I0413836

Herbal Remedies Made Easy

Your Essential Herbal Remedies Guide for Optimum Healing

Jason Neel

© 2016

Table of Contents

Chapter 1 – Introduction

Herbal Medicine is the oldest and widely spread medicine in the world, made from the plants and these medicines are used to treat different diseases and help promote optimal health conditions. It is an alternative medicine without using pharmaceutical drugs and uses herbal medicines.

There are various types of **herbal medicines** that may differ from country to country. Every country has its own nature of treatment so even though the herbs are common to all the countries, it may differ in the part that is used to prepare the medicine.

For instance, in Australia, the cultural types of medicines found are Western, Aboriginal, Auyurvedic etc., along with these cultural types, there are many other herbal treatments that may be unique in their treatments.

The medicine that is made from herbal plant or a plant part which is used for its aroma, essence or for its therapeutic properties is **Herbal Remedy**.

Herbal Remedies:

When the plants are used like a medicine. These herbal remedies are used to get relief or to prevent or cure diseases. People use these medicines to relax or get energy or even to lose weight. The herbals do not taste like medicines.

It is necessary for you to know about few facts related to the herbals before using them.

- Herbals are not controlled like medicines.

- They need not be tested before they are sold.

- Sometimes the herbal remedies may not contain the exact ingredients which are listed on the labels.

Are Herbals Safe?

Many people know that herbals are from nature, the use of herbal medicines will work more effectively than that of the normal medicines. Yet "Herbal" does not mean safe in all circumstances, if they are not taken as directed, some herbals may cause side effects as they may contains toxic when they were taken in high doses.

Read the following examples to get a clear idea about the herbal remedies.

- Take the herb of 'Kava', which is used for anxiety, insomnia and also for the symptoms of menopause. Regarding this medicine, the FDA had issued a warning as it is causing liver damage.

- People use 'St.John's Wort' for depression, birth control and other problems. This medicine in several patients caused stomach upset and for some patients caused anxiety by using this medicine.

- The bark named 'Yohimbe' is used for erectile dysfunction, but this bark in some cases increased the blood pressure, heart rate, anxiety and also many side effects. Taking this dose continuously for long periods may be dangerous, so it should be observed by the patients.

We can say that many herbs are safe and work well and cure many diseases. The only thing that one has to observe is the word 'Natural' does not mean that it is safe for everybody in all circumstances.

How to select and use the best Herbal Remedies safely?

The research says that the herbal medicines are safe and better and make you feel better and keep you fit. But before selecting and using herbal remedies the patients must choose the best medicine for their health problem.

Follow some of the tips before selecting the herbal remedies:

- Before selecting the medicine check the product description. If they give extra information that it works wonders, within seconds you will be free from the pain, or if it gives information like it is a miracle pill with which one can lose weight within no time, then you may want to proceed with caution.

- Real life experiences are not scientific research reports. It may work wonders for one person, but at the same time it may cause ill health for others. Everyone has to observe that even it was prescribed by the doctor and work excellent with patients, but it is not always same with everybody as it was not scientifically proved. It may not always provide the same results for everyone.

- Always remember to buy the herbal remedies from the certified companies. You can check the labels like "USP" verified, which have labels that are certified for their quality.

- It is not recommended the use of herbal medicines for children.

- Pregnant women should not use herbal remedies.

- Patients who have undergone any surgery should not take herbal remedies.

- Talk with your provider before you use any herbal remedies.

Herbals remedies are "Natural" medicines, they give quicker and better results. The only thing that everybody should know is that they should be taken under proper guidance and checked before use, if the medicine is suitable for their specific situation. For best results, you may want to approach your local natural health centres.

Chapter 2 – History of Herbal Remedies

Nearly 60,000 years ago, during the period of Paleolithic, people used plants as medicines. To support the claim that Paleolithic people had the knowledge of herbal medicine that researchers had gathered some of the samples from the burial sites. For instance in northern Iraq, from a 60,000 year old burial site, researchers gathered large amounts of pollen from different 8 plant species, out of which now we are using 7 plant species as herbal remedies. Even the Greeks and Romans were listed as herbalists in history.

Middle Ages

In the middle ages, Herbalism was maintained by the monks of Britain and Europe. After the advancement of education, many universities came into existence in the 11th and 12th centuries, monasteries worked as medical schools. The monks have imitated the works of Hippocrates, Dioscorides and Galen. Historians say that their gardens were well- stocked with the most common herbal medicinal plants.

At inception the Herbalism, particularly in German tribes, woman used to practice. In the 15th century after the invention of the printing press, people came to know about the herbal medicine and herbals of Dioscorides. Galen and Avicenna are produced in bulk and made available for outside the universities and the monastery. In those days people used these herbs without having any specialized skills. According to their knowledge, they gathered some of the herbs and they started using the herbs in a prescribed manner. They used to fix a dosage and followed that.

Paracelsus

Paracelsus indicated the importance of experience with the ill people and criticized against the blind faith among the physicians. Despite of his "doctrine of signatures", each and every herb got its own recognition. People came to know about the appearance, color, aroma and its medical use. The physicians in those days started treating jaundice with marigold and dandelion which has yellow flowers while pansies which look like heart shaped petals were used to cure the heart problems.

12 zodiac signs

In 1616-1654, **Nicholas Culpeper** connected the herbs to other different zodiac signs. They described which zodiac sign and planet impact is focused over the body part, that needed to be cured and prescribed a herb of the astrological sign.

William Harvey

After the promotion of the doctrine of signatures and Herbalism, slowly change began to take effect in the medical field. People like **Francis Bacon** and **William Harvey** changed the science from speculative to an regulated experimental process. This transformation of science in the initial stages did not work out properly but biological and medical sciences disconnected from the traditional Herbalism.

Herbal Medicinal Developments in 16th Century

In the year 1526, the herbals published in English were "Grete Herball", and General History of Plants and another English physician expanded the works of Nicholas Culpeper.

In Europe, the manuscripts for new medicinal plants were introduced by "The Age of exploration" and also with "Columbian Exchange" and Badianus Manuscript explained Mexican herbals.

17th Century

At inception the herbal therapeutic effects were very slow and later Paracelsus started using the chemical drugs like copper sulfate, iron, mercury, and sulfur in his medicines.

18th Century

In the 18th century, Native Americans shared their information with colonists but this information was not written and recorded until the 19th century.

19th Century

Samuel Thompson who is not a medical professional, but greatly influenced by the other medical practitioners and he is the person who introduced the formalization of pharmacology in this century which made the people to understand the action of the drugs on the human body.

Modern era

In the modern era the traditional Herbalism has officially announced as a alternative medicine in the United States.

The World Health Organization reported that nearly **80% of the people** throughout the world mostly rely on the **herbal medicines** for the primary health care. In Germany nearly **600 to 700 different plant species** are available and many are prescribed by German physicians. In South Africa, many physicians also use herbs to treat their patients.

In the 21ˢᵗ century, many medical practitioners use traditional medicine as it has a low number of side effects. Currently, there are no restrictions on the licensing or certification of herbalists in may state. So that no one is objecting to herbal use.

Chapter 3 – Kitchen Tools for Preparing Herbal Remedies

The best place for the herbalists to prepare the **herbal remedies** is the home kitchen. The kitchen is the best and the most appropriate place for the effective experimentation of herbal remedies.

In schools and colleges students are taken to the physics, biology and chemistry lab to get the practical knowledge, similarly, the herbalists need a kitchen lab and herbal garden to continue his experimentation successfully.

The herbalists need the following tools in his or her kitchen:

- To prepare the **herbal medicines**, the herbalists need bottles, jars, pots and other storage containers for mixing, boiling, stirring as well as doing whatsoever is required to complete his product.

- Remember to avoid aluminum containers as they get toxic while heating.

- It is always better to use the containers which are prepared with the stainless steel, clay pots, cast iron, ceramic containers and also glass containers.

- For measuring, the herbalists have to keep separate measuring cups for liquids, powders, and also for dried herbal materials.

- The herbalist can choose the plastic measuring cups for measuring his herbal products. They are the best suitable as they do not get rusty if we use for liquids.

- Herbal product needs scales which need not be too expensive, but the herbalist has to select the scale which measure accurately.

Few tools that you will need include:

- The **mortal and pestle** is a most important tool while preparing herbal remedies. These mortars and pestle are used when the herbalist wants to powder the barks, roots, and so on.

- **Pouring devices** like funnels also play an important role in the herbal kitchen lab. Using funnel is very easy to transfer the liquid from one container to another.

- **Grinders, Blenders, graters, knives** and other small devices are also necessary for processing the herbal remedies.

- While preparing the herbal remedies sometimes the herbalist has to check the temperature. So to check the temperature he needs a **thermometer**.

Along with the kitchen tools if the herbalist maintains a garden in his or her backyard it will be more advantageous for him/her to get the herbs freshly without losing the essence in it. If some herbs are preserved for some time there are chances to lose the essences, aroma or any important chemical substances in herbs.

To get the appropriate results, it is always better to have an herbal garden in the backyard for best results, if the weather allows in your local environment.

Chapter 4 – Health Benefits of Herbs

As the saying goes, the real wealth of any person is his health.

Yes, one has to agree with this saying. If for any reason loses money we can get it back in their lifetime. But if we neglect our health, it is irrecoverable. So everyone has to pay attention to their health to live a healthy life.

Here are simple steps on how you can add herbs to your daily diet.

- Fresh herbs you can add to your soups and also for your herbal sauces.

- Chopped, herbal leaves can be added to salads as they pass on rich necessary anti-microbial substances to your body.

- Fresh chopped herbal leaves add special flavor and taste to your vegetarian as well as non-vegetarian recipe.

- Some herbal leaves and plants are used as popular drinks.

Here is the list of herbs which are good with their health benefits.

1. *Aloe vera*

Aloe vera is a medicinal plant with rich in nutritional benefits. Aloe vera's different parts are used for different purposes. As Aloe vera is a medicinal plant it should not be consumed daily for years together.

Health Benefits

- Aloe Vera is rich in vitamins and minerals

- Aloe Vera is rich in Amino Acids and another acid like Fatty acid

- Aloe Vera is an Adaptogen

- Aloe Vera is good for digestion.

Medicinal Uses

- Aloe Vera is used in weight loss treatments.

- Aloe Vera reduces inflammation.

- This herb works like disinfectant

- Anti-biotic

- Anti-microbial

- Anti-septic

- Anti-fungal treatments.

Safety Measures

- Avoid consuming Aloe Vera internally during pregnancy. It can be used externally.

2. ***chamomile***

The herb chamomile is used for centuries. There are two types of chamomile that are used for good health (e.g., German chamomile and Roman chamomile).

Health Benefits:

- This herb can be used for irritations

- Chest cold

- Skin allergies

- Gum inflammations

- The tea prepared with this herb is best for stomach upset.

Safety Measures

- The pollen of chamomile causes allergies.

- People who are suffering with the ragweed allergy are not supposed to use this chamomile.

3. *Lavender*

The herb Lavender is originated from the mountainous Mediterranean regions of northern Africa. This herb is mostly used in skin and beauty care products. This is commonly used for its fragrances while preparing shampoos and skin creams.

Medicinal Uses

- **Lavender** oil is used as an antiseptic and anti-inflammatory and used in the burn creams and bug bite creams.

- Lavender is used to treat anxiety, insomnia and depression.

- This herb helps in treating the digestive problems, headache, hair loss and sprains, toothaches.

4. Chickweed

The scientific name of chickweed is "Stellaria media or Stellaria pubera".

The herb chickweed is a native to Europe but it is widely cultivated in other countries.

Health Benefits:

- Chickweed herb is very nutritious.

- This herb is fibrous.

- This herb consists of calcium, beta-carotene, coumarins, magnesium and zinc.

Medicinal Uses:

- The herb is used for treating skin problems.

- The herb works as an anti-inflammatory and pain reliever.

- The herb is useful to cure stomach problems.

- The herb is useful to cure liver and kidney problems.

5. *Asian Basil*

The scientific name of basil herb is "Ocimum Basilicum"

Basil is also called as "The king of the herbs and also "holy herb" in many places around the world. It is one of the ancient and most popular plants with many notable health benefits such as:

- Basila leaves are good in preventing diseases and promoting health properties.

- Basil contains **orientin and vicenin** these compounds work like anti-oxidant protection agents.

- Basila leaves contain health benefiting oils like linalool, citral, limonene etc., These oils work as anti-inflammatory and anti-bacterial properties.

- The basil herb contains low level calories and is cholesterol free. So it is one of the richest sources to get nutrients, minerals, and vitamins to maintain good health conditions.

Medicinal Uses

- Basil herb oil works as an anti-infective against bacteria like Staphylococcus.

- Tea prepared with basil leaves gives relief from nausea and performs anti-septic functions.

6. Burdock Root/Burdock Plant

The Scientific name of burdock root is "Arctium Lappa." Burdock Root is used as a vegetable and a medicinal herb. In Japan, this root is known as **'gobo'**. This root was cultivated in large scale and in many parts of the globe.

Some of the health benefits of burdock roots are:

- The young roots which have enormous compounds that are used as anti-oxidant, prevents diseases and improves health conditions.

- Burdock root is rich in **potassium** and low in sodium.

- This root contains **vitamin E** and **vitamin C**.

- This root contains minerals like **manganese, iron and magnesium.**

Medicinal Uses

- Burdock herb is used as a **blood purifier**.

- This herb is used to treat **skin problems**.

- Burdock seeds are used for **chest ailments** and also for throat infections.

- This herb stems and leaves are also used as an **appetite stimulant**.

7. Ginger Herb and Root

The scientific name of ginger is *'Zingiber Officinale'*

Its benefits include:

- Ginger root is used as **anti-inflammatory, anti-flatulent** and also like **anti-microbial** properties.

- Ginger herb contains benefitting oils like shogaol, farnesene which are used to relieve from **nausea, migraine headache** and it can be used as anti-bacterial substance.

- This herb is rich in **potassium, manganese, magnesium** and **copper**.

Medicinal Uses:

- If we boil ginger root along with lemon or orange, the liquid concentrate is used an herbal drink to cure **common cold, sore throat and cough.**

- In Ayurvedic medicine the taste of the ginger covers the bitterness taste and allows the patient to take it freely.

- This root increases **motility of the gastrointestinal** tract.

- It reduces **migraine.**

8. Garlic

The scientific name of Garlic is "Allium Sativum." Garlic has a good recognition in medicinal properties and in culinary uses. The root contains phyto-nutrient substances and reported as the best medicine to cure **infections.**

Health Benefits

- Garlic cloves contain **minerals, vitamins, anti-oxidants**

- Garlic is rich source in **potassium, calcium, manganese, zinc and selenium.**

Medicinal Uses

- Garlic cloves can be used to cure **cold, cough** and **bronchitis**.

- Garlic oil can be used as external applicant for **ring worm and skin infections.**

- It works as an **anti-diabetic**

- **Anti-microbial**

- It lowers the **cholesterol.**

9. Coriandrum/Coriander leaves

It is a perennial herb and grows if it is cultivated in fertile soil, well draining facility, and favorable climate.

Health Benefits

- The coriander leaves are rich in **potassium, calcium, manganese, iron and magnesium.**

- It is also rich **in vitamin C**, **vitamin A** and **folic acid**.

- The coriander leaves are herbal sources for **vitamin K.**

Medicinal Uses

- The leaves are used in **deodorants**

- Helps with digestion

- Stimulant and stomach ache

- Analgesic and in fungicidal medicines.

- Coriander leaves are used in cooking in soups ,sauces, vegetarian and non vegetarian dishes.

- In salads

10. Borage

Borage is a stemmed plant with bristly hairs and grows in Europe and in some parts of Asia. The leaves of Borage are used in salads. The leaves of Borage become tougher, larger and tastes better as it gets older.

Health Benefits

- The Borage herb contains gamma-linolenic acid which is a powerful anti-oxidant and immune booster.

- This herb contains wound healing power and also acts as an anti-viral substance.

- This herb is rich in **Vitamin A, Vitamin C, iron, calcium, potassium, manganese, copper, zinc, potassium and also magnesium.**

Medicinal Uses

- The Borage is used to cure **arthritis, dermatitis** and to relief **pre-menstrual pain.**

- This herb is also used in traditional medicines to improve the breast milk in the nursing mothers.

- A word of caution of safety with this herb and not be over consumed as it cause significant health implications including kidney problem.

11. **Leaf-celery/Celery stalks**

Celery herb starts flowering from the second year. The Chinese celery appears with thin and hollow stalks. The important aspect is the stalks of this herb are more flavor and the seeds look like cumin seeds in dark brown color and have a strong flavor and aroma.

Health Benefits

- The Celery herb is rich in **vitamin A, vitamin K, vitamin C, Folic acid** and this herb is a very source of minerals like **potassium, sodium, calcium, and magnesium.**

- Celery leaf, roots and stalks can be used in salads and stews.

- This herb is used in preparing soups and sauces.

Medicinal Uses

- Celery reduces **blood pressure and indigestion**

- This herb removes excess water from the body.

- This herb works as an **anti-inflammatory agent.**

Safety measures

- This herb is not safe to be used by the pregnant women.

- Sometimes it causes anaphylactic reactions, so sensitive individuals are not supposed to have this herb.

- Too much of celery herb may cause **stomach pain** and **constipation**.

12. *Epazote*

Epazote can be grown annually. This herb needs to have sandy soil, more sunlight and well draining facilities.

Health Benefits

- This herb is rich in **protein**, **fiber** and **phyto nutrients.**

- The young leaves of this herb are rich in **folic acid**.

- This herb has small amounts of **vitamin A and anti- oxidants**.

Medicinal Uses

- The Epazote herb works works for the **intestinal ailments, ulcers, indigestion,** and **cramps.**

- This herb is good for **stomach pain.**

Safety Measures

- It is safe to use this herb in small quantities.

- It is not safe for the pregnant women.

- Over dosage may affect the heart and nervous system so use with extra caution.

13.   Lemongrass herb/Lemongrass stem

Lemongrass scientific name is "Cymbopogon citrates." This herb belongs to the grass family and is found in Sri Lanka, Thailand, Vietnam, Malaysia, Cambodia and Indonesia.

Health Benefits

- The lemongrass herb contains **minerals, vitamins and disease preventing properties.**

- This herb contains only small amounts of **vitamin A and C.**

- This herb is rich in **potassium, zinc, calcium, iron, magnesium** etc.

- Lemongrass is one the ingredients in **sea foods, meat and poultry**.

- It is used in soups, curries and fries also.

Medicinal Uses

- The lemongrass controls **heart rate**.

- This herb controls **blood pressure.**

- This herb is used to flavor the herbal tea powder.

- Lemongrass oil is used to relieve **headache, body-aches, nervous exhaustion** and to relieve in stress.

14. *Peppermint*

Peppermint originated in Europe. It grows in shady places. This plant does not produce seeds. There are nearly 20 varieties of peppermint herbs with different colors, fragrance, and flavor.

Health Benefits

- Peppermint is rich in **vitamin C, vitamin E and vitamin K**

- Peppermint is rich in **potassium**, **calcium**, **manganese** and **magnesium.**

Medicinal Uses

- This herb is used for bad breath like mouthwash, tooth paste and in chewing gums.

- This herb is also used in cough syrups, mouth and throat infection medicines and nasal inhalers.

Chapter 5 – How to Use Herbs to Stay Healthy and Disease-free

Herbalist and acupuncture physicians say that **herbal *medicine*** has a long history, which are used for thousands of years. Especially **kitchen *medicine*** is very much popularized and the natural treatments have not changed and have improved as global choices are increasing. Here are few instructions on how to add the herbs to your recipe and make you stay healthy.

Let us have a glance at his valuable instructions:

1. **Rosemary**

   ➤ Herb **'Rosemary'** which is a strong flavored herb can be added to your regular diet. This herb helps prevent damages to the blood vessels, indigestion, reduces muscle and joint pains. Rosemary can be used in potatoes, meat, pan juices and chicken.

2. **Parsley**

Several studies found that this herb help inhibit the growth of the cancer, prevents heart problems, and lowers blood pressure. This herb can be added to your diet as a chopped garnish and can be added to the chicken creole.

3. **Cinnamon**

By using cinnamon twigs one can be free from gastrointestinal disturbances, diarrhea, and controls type 2 blood sugar levels. As cinnamon acts as antibiotic and anti-inflammatory it can be added to all curries for taste and flavor.

4. **Sage**

Sage is used in many beauty creams. This is a wonderful herb which fights against early aging. If you add it your diet then no need to buy any beauty creams which fights against early aging.

To be free from memory loss one can add this sage in their routine diet. It can be grown in your backyard and can add to your diet.

5. Cilantro

Cilantro is rich in **iron** which is most important for our body. Our body takes metals and sends the excess of metals through tissues. So cilantro helps in sending out the excess metals.

6. Dill

Dill is a flavorful herb. By using dill one can control the diseases like inflammation, indigestion, respiratory disorders, diarrhea and dysentery.

Dill can be used in many cuisines, used in yogurt, topping soups, sour creams, topping for cooked potatoes. In the summer, chopped dill can be added to buttermilk for better taste. It can be used in sandwiches and salads.

7. Thyme

Those who are suffering from bronchitis, low blood pressure, cough, infections can use thyme to boosts their mood, acts as disinfect etc.,

Thyme can be used in cooking. The leaves and edible parts of the plant and can be used for cooking. Thyme can be added with all other vegetables. So add thyme to your regular diet and be disease free.

As herbs contain minerals, vitamins, and other necessary substances which are very important for the human body, they should be added to your regular diet.

Chapter 6 – How to Grow Your Own Herbs

Based on the soil and weather conditions, one can have their own preferences in a backyard herb garden.

Location: Select place where you want to start a garden. Remove all the grass and unwanted material from the location. It is important to see that your garden needs at least 7 hours of sunlight a day.

- Select the suitable plants for your climate. While choosing the plants to your garden, remember that they have to suit your climate. If your soil doesn't in condition do a fair planning with other sources such as raised beds or pot gardening. For raised beds and container gardening you need more planning because they require more maintaining optimal conditions to raise the good growth.

These are the basic things you need to start a backyard herbal garden.

Herb Garden: If your location and your climate suits best you can start an herb garden.

- Select your required herbs.

- Till the garden.

- On the top of the soil, shovel compost and mix it thoroughly.

- Plant the seeds.

- Water them daily

First decide the herbs what you want to grow, then make sure that they are suitable for your climatic conditions. Select the herbs which you can cook regularly and plant the same in the garden for regular use. Here is the list of some herbs which can be grown in your herbal garden.

Information related to, how to plant, care, harvest and use the herbs which you are selecting to plant in the garden.

❖ **Basil:** If you have selected basil herb in your garden, then just remember to pinch the flowers of the Basil herb to increase the flavor. It also increases the density of the stem.

- When you decide to harvest the Basil herb, remove few leaves from each stem.

- You can use this Basil herb in salads, sandwiches, soups, sauces, pizza and also in making pesto.

❖ **Parsley:** This herb needs more patience to germinate as it takes three to four weeks extra period.

- This herb can be harvested by cutting the stalks above the ground level. This in return encourages the further growth.

- Parsley's leaves and stalks can be used in salads, soups and also in dishes like Tabouli.

❖ **Rosemary:** Rosemary can be carefully planted. This herb does not need more water.

- This herb is very easy to use. When you need it, you can cut off the stem and use freshly for cooking.

- This herb has many medicinal uses and is culinary.

❖ **Mint:** This is an invasive plant which can be grown in the herb garden.

- You can use the sprigs as and when you need.

- As it is very versatile, you can use mint in drinks, desserts, you can also chew it for flavor, and it can be used in salads.

❖ **Thyme:** To plant thyme in your garden, you can germinate a seed or buy a mature plant. This is very suitable for the drier soils and very easy to care.

- You can take off the pieces of the stem when you need to use.

- This Thyme can be used in meat, soups and stews.

Acquire the basic information and follow suitable steps to start and protect your garden from pest and fertilizers and enjoy the fun in gardening. A planned and well organized herb garden provides you self-employed satisfaction, as gardening involves exercise you will be healthy.

Having an herb garden makes you healthy by providing rich nutrition items.

Chapter 7 – Buying Herbs at Your Local Store

Herbs have a long history in cooking, cosmetics, and medicinal purposes. These days, they are very much popularized around the world as people want to seek a natural and healthy lifestyle.

Herbal growth has increased intensely in recent years. As the herbs contain many health benefits and medicinal values today, many add the herbs in their regular diet. New research has proven that herbs are the alternative to expensive pharmaceutical drugs.

People are aware of the uses of the herbs, ultimately started using them, and now started in search of the fresh herbs which can be used in their cooking. If you can grow them in your garden that is the best way to have access to fresh herbs at your finger tips. Many people lack the resources to grow the Herbs mainly, because of lack of time and may not have suitable place to grow them.

How to select the best herbs to buy at the local markets?

The first thing is to select the vendor who is selling fresh herbs. Only buy the dry herbs if you have limited options in your area.

What you have to look for, when you are buying the herbs in the local market?

- When you are buying the herbs, first observe its color. Most of the herbs should be green in color and some herbs in dark green in color.

- Check the herb whether it is fresh or not. If it is fresh it should get the strong aroma. Herbs that are with no smell or weak smell are not so fresh herbs and are considered old.

- If there is no market nearby where you can obtain the fresh herbs, try to purchase them in the nearby market and store them to use according to your convenience.

- Store your herbs in the recycled jars, quart jars or use tight lid jars to preserve your herbs.

Many herbs are available throughout the year, some herbs are only seasonal. Gather the information related to the seasonal herbs and try to purchase them in the as use according to your requirement.

Chapter 8 – The Top 10 Herbs Must Have Handy

Herbs and spices which have a long history are incredibly substantial and are added to our regular usage directly or indirectly. Many of the herbs are used in the cosmetics and in medical purposes along with their culinary use. Research has proven that herbs have remarkable health benefits, so they should be added to our regular diet to stay healthy and disease-free.

These are the top ten herbs and spices which have proven to have health benefits:

Cinnamon: This is a well-known spice, as we will use in all sorts of recipes and especially non-vegetarian dishes. This spice has a medical property that is the compound which is present in cinnamon is "cinnamaldehyde", which has an **antioxidant activity**. Some health benefits of adding cinnamon to your diet include:

- Reduce **blood pressure**

- Effective to **control the blood sugar levels**

- Anti-inflammatory

- Reduces the risk of **heart diseases**

- Beneficial effects on **Neurodegenerative problems**

- Fights **bacteria other infections like fungal**

Sage: Sage is a Latin word which means "to save." Obviously it shows its potency in the middle age as this herb has a strong reputation and was used against plague. Some of its outstanding health benefits include:

- It improves brain function and increases the memory power.

- A thorough research on 50 patients reported that sage works wonder for the "Alzheimer's disease", where it showed a decrease in the level of acetylcholine in the brain, helping in managing the disease.

- Sage improves the memory power.

Basil: Basil is a sacred herb in many cultures. Research shows that it has many medicinal functions. Some of its health benefits include:

- Improves the immune cells in the blood.
- Prevents the growth of bacteria which causes ill health.
- Reduces the blood sugar levels.
- Reduces anxiety.

Cayenne: Cayenne is used in spicy dishes and has so many health benefits, including:

- Helps in weight loss.
- Reduces appetite.
- Burns fat

Thyme: It has many effective health benefits, including:

- Fights depression

- Helps eliminate nail fungus

- Helps with hair loss

- Helps with headache

- Eliminates snoring

Ginger Herb and Root: Heath benefits of ginger include:

- Anti-inflammatory, anti-flatulent and also like anti-microbial properties.

- Treatment for shogaol, farnesene which are used to relieve from nausea, migraine headache and it can be used as anti-bacterial substance.

- This herb is rich in potassium, manganese, and magnesium and also copper.

Garlic Bulbs*: Garlic has a good recognition in medicinal properties. The root or bulb contains phyto-nutrient substances and reported as the best medicine to cure infections.

Fenugreek: It is used in Ayurvedic medicines. Human studies stated that one gram of Fenugreek everyday reduces the blood sugar levels. It functions as a insulin for diabetic patients.

Turmeric: Turmeric poweder has its own significance. This spice is used regularly in the cooking. If you pinch turmeric powder in your dish it will give it a nice aroma and color for your dish. It is rich in curcumin, which acts as a powerful antioxidant. Turmeric powder reduces the risk of heart diseases.

Dandelion herb/Dandelion leaves: Dandelion originated from the Central Asia. This herb is very hardy which grows everywhere. Dandelion is used to treat gall bladder problems. It can also be used as a appetite stimulant.

Chapter 9 – Herbal Remedies for the top 100 Ailments

Ailment	Herbs
1.Headache	Butterbur, ginger, caffeine, coriander, almonds, feverfew
2.Asthma	Butterbur, ginger, mustard oil, figs, coffee
3.Fever	Butterbur, apple cider vinegar, garlic, raisins, basil, ginger, water
4.Cough	Butterbur, honey, gargle with salt, thyme tea, black pepper
5.Gastrointestinal problems	Butterbur, peppermint, lemon balm, ginger, fennel seeds, dandelion
6.Toothaches	Peppermint, salt water, garlic, cloves, onion, vanilla extract
7.Spasms	Peppermint, mullein, hops, drink water, stretch, passion flower, celery seed
8.Nausea	Peppermint, ginger, fresh lemon, dry toast, rest
9.Stomach	Ginger, caffeine, chamomile

Ailment	Herbs
pain	tea, mint, lemon water, ginger tea
10. Arthritis	Ginger, horseradish, turmeric, aloe vera, eucalyptus, green tea
11. Cold and flu	Ginger tea, honey, garlic, radish, chicken soup, steam, goral with salt
12. Neurological problems	Ginger, wild carrot, Indian gooseberry, cinnamon, turmeric
13. High blood pressure	Caffeine, basil, cinnamon, cardamom, flaxseed, garlic,
14. Sexually transmitted diseases	Peppermint tea, bicarbonate soda, cranberry juice, lemon juice
15. Irritable bowl syndrome	Yogurt, peppermint tea, ginger, exercise
16. Inflammation	Caffeine, coriander, dandelion, turmeric, extra virgin olive oil
17. Skin damage	Caffeine, avocado, coconut, egg white mask, honey, yogurt, aloe vera
18. Kidney	Caffeine, horseradish,

Ailment	Herbs
disease	dandelion, parsley juice, green tea, apple cider vinegar
19.Heart problems	Valerian, garlic, hawthorn, Chinese hibiscus, turmeric, cayenne
20.Tremors	Valerian, essential oils, omega3,
21.Anxiety	Valerian, hops, chamomile, omeg3, lavender essential oil, exercise or walk
22.Fatigue	Coriander, lavender, dandelion, ginseng, lemon, yoga, meditation
23.Nerve pain	Coriander, ginger, turmeric, acupuncture, massage
24.Stress	Lavender, slow and deep breezing, meditation, chamomile tea, basil, dark chocolate, massage, sauna,
25.Muscle and joint pain	Rosemary, ginger, turmeric, magnesium, extra virgin olive oil, dandelions, molasses, exercise
26.Memory problems	Rosemary, almonds, black seed, Indian goose berry, fish oil,
27.Liver	Rosemary, cumin seeds,

Ailment	Herbs
ailments	Carmon seeds, garlic, papaya seeds, turmeric
28.Migraines	Rosemary, mullein, magnesium, feverfew, peppermint, lavender, essential oils, water
29.Nervous disorder	Rosemary, chamomile, ashwagandha, passion flower, green tea, black tea, lavender, kava
30.Bladder infection	Horseradish, drink water, cranberry juice, parsley juice, celery seeds, cucumber,
31.Joint pain	Horseradish, turmeric, ginger, oil oil
32.Muscle strains	Horseradish, ice, Epsom salt, apple cider
33. Wounds	Honeysuckle, clean, coconut oil, turmeric, aloe vera
34.Red eyes	Cold water, rosewater, cucumber, tea bag,
35.Virus	Honeysuckle, garlic, ginger, elderberry
36.Sores	Honeysuckle, olive oil, baking soda, chamomile tea, sage,

Ailment	Herbs
	coconut oil, honey, aloe vera, salt water
37.Infections	Honeysuckle, garlic, onion, grapefruit extract, horseradish, citrus fruits, raw honey, cinnamon
38.Diarrhea	Mullein, black tea, blackberries, yogurt
39.Pain relieving	Yarrow, ginseng, kava kava, valerian root, St. John's Wort, essential oil
40.Anti anxiety	Yarrow, chamomile, passion flower, lavender
41.Ulcer	Bananas, coconut, cabbage, fenugreek
42.Vomiting	Teaberry, evodia, honey, ginger, rice water, mint
43.Sleep problems	Hops, valerian, cherries, chamomile, bananas, exercise, drink water, lavender
44.Cholestrol	Hops, hawthorn, flaxseed, fish oil, garlic
45.Neuralgia	Hops, hot and cold packs, essential oils, St. John's Wort tea, celery juice

Ailment	Herbs
46.Cramps	Hops, ginger, fennel, Chinese herbs
47.Blood pressure	Evodia, hibiscus, reduce salt, coconut water, fish oil, Hawthorn,
48.Heart problems	Rosemary, garlic, ginger, Hawthorn, turmeric, cayenne,
49.Hypertension	Parsley, garlic, fish oil, hibiscus, dark chocolate, magnesium, green coffee extract
50.Alzheimer disease	Sage, coconut oil, cinnamon, lemon balm, sun, fish oil, ginseng, cat's claw, cross word
51.Immune function	Basil, Echinacea, ginseng, garlic, bell papers, ginger, turmeric
52.Weightloss	Cayenne, honey and lemon, green tea, parsley, apple cider vinegar, curry leaves, cinnamon tea, ginseng
53.Appetite	Cayenne, coriander, garlic, cardamom, ginger, black paper, dandelion, arugula
54.Blood sugar	Fenugreek, cinnamon, Indian Gooseberry, mango leaves, garlic, blueberries, apple cider

Ailment	Herbs
	vinegar, black coffee,
55.Insect bites	Garlic, baking soda, aloe vera, raw honey
56. Bruises	Comfrey leaves, cabbage, cayenne pepper, lavender oil, aloe vera, garlic
57.Acid reflex	Angelica, caraway, clown's mustard plant, licorice
58.Gingivitis	Turmeric, aloe vera, salt, baking soda, lemon juice, sage, oil pulling
59.Irritable bowl syndrome	Peppermint, fennel, ginger, chamomile, caraway, anise, oregano
60.Pink eye	Tulsi, aloe vera, turmeric, neem oil
61.Poison ivy	Aloe vera, organic goldenseal, apple cider vinegar, oatmeal paste, banana peel, cucumber, watermelon
62.Yeast infection	Garlic, yogurt, coconut, cranberry, tea tree oil, cotton underwear
63.Backpain	Cranberry juice, barley water, yoga, pipsissewa, stretching,

Ailment	Herbs
	exercise
64. Pinworms	Garlic, grapefruit extract, coconut, carrot
65.Forstbite	Lavender, aloe vera, tea bag, liquids, olive oil, mustard oil, ginger
66.Cellulite	Tomatoes paste, ginko biloba, dry brushing, coffee scrub, omega3, coconut oil, green tea, apple cider vinegar, cayenne pepper, gelatin
67.Dandruff	Fenugreek, methi, aspirin, aloe vera, apple cider vinegar, baking soda, Listerine, sun, lemons
68.Diarrhea	Psyllium seeds, carrots, yogurt, ginger, fenugreek seeds, bananas, apple cider vinegar, chamomile tea
69.Hay fever	Chamomile, ginger, peppermint, honey, apple cider vinegar, turmeric
70.Morning sickness	Ginger, peppermint tea, lemon wedges, fennel seed
71.Nose	Cayenne, pinch the nose, apple cider vinegar, cold compress,

Ailment	Herbs
bleeding	onion, nettle
72.Intestinal worms	Garlic, coconut, unripe papaya, carrot, pumpkin, turmeric
73. Hair split ends	Methi, eggs, avocado, bananas, papaya, honey, coconut oil, chamomile tea
74.Sunburn	Aloe vera, coconut oil, milk, sunflower seeds, cucumber, teabag
75.Dry skin	Aloevera, olive oil, milk cream, honey, yogurt, coconut oil, oatmeal
76.Stretch marks	Aloevera, egg whites, lemon juice, potato juice, almond oil and sugar, drink water, coco butter, lavender oil
77.Periodont al disease	Aloe vera, oil pulling, sage, garlic and turmeric paste, mustard oil, salt water
78.Depression	St. John's Wort, omega3, saffron, green tea, meditation, exercise, eat nutritious food, chamomile tea
79. Sore throat	Gargle with salt water, garlic, marshmallow, cayenne, baking

Ailment	Herbs
	soda
80. Ear infection	Garlic, salt, basil, apple cider vinegar, olive oil, warm water, tea tree oil, basil
81. Sprains	Compression, ice, turmeric, garlic, olive oil, onion, cabbage, ginger
82.Stiff muscles	Crampbark, apple cider vinegar, coconut oil, massage, exercise, rest
83.Diuretic	Dandelion, hawthorn, horsetail extract, green tea, parsley, hibiscus
84.Motion sickness	Ginger, peppermint, fennel, rosemary, basil, parsley
85. Dry lips	St. John's wort, honey, sugar, coconut oil, milk cream, mustard oil
86.Ease muscle tension	Skullcap, acupuncture, relaxation, yoga, exercise, cherry juice, hot bath
87. Dry mouth	Drink fluids, cayenne, fennel seed, oil pulling, aloe vera
88.Osteoarthritis	Willow bark, exercise, ice or heat therapies, ginger,

Ailment	Herbs
	turmeric, cinnamon
89. Stimulate digestion	Yellow dock, ginger, yogurt, peppermint, sweet potatoes, avocados, oats, dandelions
90.Eczema	Jojoba oil, coconut oil, teabags, omega3, lavender essential oil, sun
91.Skin itching	Baking soda, lemon, oatmeal, apple cider vinegar, honey,
92.Black circles under eyes	Cucumber, potatoes, green tea bags, rose water, almond oil, milk, tomatoes, mint leaves, buttermilk pate, avocado, meditation
93.Dengue fever	Coriander, basil leaves, fenugreek, neem leaves, basil leaves, papaya juice
94. Excessive sweating	Herbal tea, tomato juice, natural vinegar, witch hazel, potatoes, coconut oil, grapes,
95.Hair loss	Methi seed powder, Arandi oil, fenugreek, onion juice, aloe vera, licorice root, rosemary, jojoba oil, coconut, henna, Indian gooseberry
96.Kidney	Dandelion root, kidney beans,

Ailment	Herbs
infection/stones	horsetail
97.Wrist tendinitis	Ice, acupuncture, ginger, cinnamon, berries, pineapple, coconut water
98.Thyroid	Lyceum berry, marine phytoplankton, bugleweed, lemon balm, broccoli, omega3
99.Menopause	Black cohosh, dong quai, kava, fruit and veggies, avocado, water, red clover, ginseng
100. knee pain	Turmeric, ginger, dandelion leaves

Conclusion

Thank you again for buying this book!

I hope this book was able to help you learn about the many herbal and medicinal remedies. Herbs I have presented in this book can be easily incorporated in your healthy food eating habits as they add special flavor to your foods. The herbs also contain anti-microbial substances which protects us from free radicals. If you add the herbs to your daily diet, they in return will not only add special favor but also improve our immune system from various diseases. The top 100 ailments presented can be treated the list of herbs and natural foods to treat them and remain healthy and disease-free without pharmaceutical drugs by making simple everyday herbs and foods part of our healthy lifestyles.

Finally, if you found the information in this book helpful, please let your friends and colleagues know your thoughts by leaving a review for this book on Amazon. I would also greatly appreciate your feedback on the book.

Thank you and to your good health and success!

Regards,

Jason Neel